Conquer And Control

Your Smoking Habits

Alan Fensin

Published by Burlington Books Div.
Burlington National Inc.
Box 841, Mandeville, LA 70470
United States of America
www.conquerandcontrol.com

Disclaimer
	All matters regarding your health require medical supervision. The ideas, procedures and suggestions contained in this book are not intended as a substitute for advice, consultation or treatment by licensed practitioners. By reading or using the information contained in this book, you are accepting responsibility for your own health and health decisions and expressly release the author and the publisher from any and all liability, loss and consequences whatsoever, including those arising from negligence.
	The information in this book comes from highly regarded sources. Although reasonable efforts were made to publish reliable information, the author and the publisher assume no responsibility for the material or any consequences of its use.

Library of Congress Control Number: 2014911730

ISBN 978-1-57706-668-2
Printed in the United States of America.

What people are saying about *Conquer and Control*

Conquer and Control isn't some feel-good, just-be-positive stuff. It is a logical and practical formula that you can apply to change your habits. — Joseph Keene

A pioneering and invaluable work about how to change smoking habits. — Chester Imperato

This book offers indispensable practical methods to change some really bad habits. — Bill Malone

The *Conquer and Control* strategies are much more powerful than just using willpower. Properly executed, the *Conquer and Control* principles will drastically improve your life. — Allen Brusiewski

If you want to stop smoking, this book is invaluable. Get it and use it! — Jim Locke

Buy this book. You won't be disappointed — it will change your life. — Robert LaPierre

Fensin boils down years of research to give us proven methods to change our destructive smoking habits. — Bob Porter

This book takes us on a tour of our subconscious mind and shows us how to exert conscious control to change it and stop our smoking habits. — Bert Phillips

Lots of books tell you what you should do, but this book shows you how to do it. — Raymond Cuomo

This is a fascinating look into the workings of the subconscious brain and how to exert control over its vast potential to control our lives. — Sam Lottel

Packed full of insights to changing smoking habits, this book is well written and highly recommended. — Ed Jensen

Thank you for this book. It is a well-researched and effective way to change smoking addictions. This book should be required reading in every school.
— Clint Cardoza

Contents

Introduction		7
Chapter 1	**Smoking**	9
Chapter 2	**Habit Change**	23
	How Habits Work	26
	Cue, Action, Reward	27
	Belief	34
	Summary of Chapter	37
Chapter 3	**Subconscious Mind**	39
	Conscious Mind	50
	Subconscious Mind Control,	52
	Seven Step Subconscious Session	57
	Summary of Chapter	65
Conclusion		71
About the Author		73

Introduction

Congratulations on your decision to quit smoking. It's amazing how many people blame society or someone else not only for their smoking problems, but also for the other problems in their life. They blame their lot in life on upbringing, family, health, bad luck, lack of money or 'the man' (usually the government, their spouse or their boss). You will learn in this book that the external world does exert influence over your habit formation, but you can regain control at any time you choose. In fact, playing the blame game gives you the illusion that you have less power than you really have. You can continue to blame someone else, or you can learn to take responsibility for your smoking addiction and learn how to change. Your life can be so much easier then you imagine.

When people discover that they that they are addicted to nicotine and don't know how to stop smoking, they sometimes lose their self-respect and replace it with self-disgust or even self-loathing. When they finally manage to become free of the addiction, they often feel they are finally a success and their real lives have finally begun.

Major change of any kind in your life is often fearful. For many people, the mere thought of giving up their cigarettes can fill them with fear. You may have a goal of one day giving up your addiction, but today may not be the day. You may have previously tried to 'quit', but after much hard work and effort were unsuccessful.

The most important thing in having a happy, addiction-free life is to make habits your friends and allies instead of your enemies and destroyers. Changing an undesirable habit can be difficult if you do not understand how to do it. This is because your habits are implanted deep in your subconscious mind. Trying to fight or resist a bad habit without knowing how often just makes the habit more powerful. The key to changing habits is to use the methods of habit change and subconscious mind control given in the final two chapters of this book.

The *Conquer and Control* method is real. It is different than anything you have tried before. If you truly want to break your nicotine addiction, this method will allow you to do so. It works because it combines the latest science on habit change with some of the latest technology on subconscious mind control. Taken together, you will have the tools you need to take your life back. There is nothing else like it. There is no other book like this one.

Chapter one gives you some basic information about nicotine addiction. It addresses the problems—both mental and physical—that addiction can present and provides you with the basics of how to approach those problems.

Chapter two explains how habits work. Once you understand the makeup of your life-destroying smoking habit, you can determine which part of the habit to change.

Chapter three teaches you the tools you need in order to use your conscious mind to reprogram your subconscious mind. You will use this reprogramming to change your smoking habit.

Together, the three chapters of this book give you everything you need to change your destructive smoking habit.

A good life requires enough control of your mind to adjust the factors that can lead to positive change in your life. That is what this book is about.

> You are always free to change your mind and choose a different future, or a different past. — Richard Bach

Chapter One
Cigarettes Addiction

> If somebody invented cigarettes today, the government would not legalize them. — Loni Anderson

I am sure everyone already knows that cigarettes are bad for their health. In America, every cigarette pack has a large, prominently displayed health warning citing lung cancer, heart disease, emphysema and other ailments. Many other countries have even stronger cigarette health warnings.

So most people know that smoking is a risk and really want to quit. About three quarters of American smokers say they want to quit and believe that one day they will quit.

But it is not that easy to be free of nicotine addiction. Often people try smoking fewer cigarettes in the hope that they can eventually get to zero. This frequently works for a little while, but the problem is that it is usually not a permanent solution. This is because the nicotine addiction and smoking habits are still there and most people eventually lose their willpower and return to heavy usage.

If you have tried to stop smoking, you probably found that nicotine withdrawal is difficult; that you could stop for a week or so, but not forever. Or perhaps you never tried to quit. Either way, the process in this book will allow you to become smoke free forever.

About half of all America smokers actually try to quit every year, but most just use will power or nicotine replacement therapy, such as electronic cigarettes or nicotine gum. The vast majority of these people start smoking again. With the subconscious habit change methods in this book, you will be able to quit smoking and stay smoke free forever.

> People always come up to me and say that my smoking is bothering them... Well, it's killing me! — Wendy Liebman

There are two fundamental reasons why people continue to smoke. First is the addictive quality of nicotine, which is a very powerful drug. It very easy to unknowingly develop a physical addiction to nicotine. If most people had realized when they first picked up a cigarette that they would become hooked on them, they likely would not have started in the first place.

The second reason is the ritual habit of smoking. Most people are attached to various habits, such as needing a cigarette at certain times (including taking a break from work, after a meal, or after sex). In addition to the nicotine addiction, you have developed a smoking habit.

This smoking habit is entirely subconscious. You don't think about how you take the cigarette out of the pack and light a fire to begin the ritual. You don't think about how you hold the cigarette or how you put something in your mouth to suck. You don't think about how to inhale the smoke. It is a habit. You are busy doing something with your hands and mouth and the whole thing is a habit that must be changed for you do become smoke free.

Additionally, cigarette companies spend billions of dollars every year and use various advertising venues to keep your subconscious mind thinking that cigarettes give you status, sophistication, and confidence, and that they relax you when you are nervous. These advertisements typically try to create a subconscious association between cigarettes and images of attractive, athletic people climbing mountains, riding horses etc. The object is to subconsciously pair cigarettes with health, sexuality, romance and good times.

> The true face of smoking is disease, death and horror—not the glamour and sophistication the pushers in the tobacco industry try to portray. — David Byrne

Once you understand these that both of these factors combine to keep you addicted, you can develop the power to change them and quit smoking.

It should be no surprise that cigarette manufactures don't want you to quit smoking. In addition to their commercials, many actually add flavors and additional nicotine to their cigarettes to achieve maximum addictive potential so you stay hooked. They actually have registered patents about how to control nicotine levels by extracting nicotine from tobacco stems with various chemicals and adding the nicotine to the tobacco leaf.

> The best way to stop smoking is to just stop... no ifs, ands or butts. — Edith Zittler

Nicotine is the drug in cigarettes that gets you addicted. It is a very addictive drug and just one cigarette is all it takes for many people to become addicted. In America, slightly more than half of the population has smoked at some point during their life.

Another word for addiction is dependence. Today, approximately twenty percent of the adult American population is dependent on cigarettes and smokes at least one each day. However, that number is decreasing.

Smoking the cigarette is the drug delivery system that uses your lungs to put the nicotine drug directly and very quickly into your blood stream. Within seconds your withdraw symptoms disappear and you feel much more relaxed. This immediate relief from your withdrawal nervousness is what makes the cigarette so addictive.

Among the other dangerous additives in most cigarettes is saltpeter (potassium nitrate). Saltpeter is the main ingredient in black gunpowder. Its purpose in cigarettes is to keep them burning so you do not have to constantly relight it. However, in some people, saltpeter can cause kidney disease, high blood pressure, heart problems, gastroenteritis and anemia. The combination of nicotine and saltpeter makes smoking the number one cause of preventable death in America.

Of course, the carbon monoxide, tar, nicotine and thousands of combustion byproducts in the cigarette trigger various cancers, heart diseases, immune disease, obstructive pulmonary disease, various other lung diseases, and more. Millions of smokers die just from smoking. Smoking has also been correlated with premature aging of the skin, a weakened immune system and even erectile dysfunction. Nicotine from cigarettes is a drug that has very few good effects but has many painful, horrible, and deadly side effects. It is truly the main problem with smoking.

Carbon monoxide (CO) is a poisonous gas even in small concentrations, and cigarette smoke contains very high levels of it. Carbon monoxide should not be confused with carbon dioxide (CO_2), which is a harmless gas in all but the highest concentrations.

When you inhale carbon monoxide it enters your blood stream and permanently binds to the hemoglobin in your red blood cells. This prevents those cells from carrying oxygen to all of the various parts of your body. The resulting decrease in oxygenation is one of the main factors that causes smokers to have increased rates of cardiovascular disease as well as other problems throughout their body.

The good news is that when you quit smoking, it only takes a week or so for your carbon monoxide and blood chemistry return to normal levels. This is because your body is constantly making new red blood cells and disposing of the old ones. However, the residual damage to your body can take much longer to heal.

So if everyone already knows the dangers of smoking why am I mentioning it again? Your mind probably rationalized the dangers long ago. "Some smokers live their entire lives without problems," you thought, "so it probably won't happen to me." However, the odds are very much against you. You will eventually have health problems. Look at the negatives again; dying from some of the complications from smoking can be a painful and terrible way to go.

After being smoke free for 15 years, your risk of heart disease is the same as a non-smoker. Your risk of cancer and some of the other common problems decreases sharply; not as low as someone who never smoked in their life, but much better than someone who still smokes. The sooner you stop, the better your odds for a healthy life.

> Smoking sucks! The one thing I would say to my kid is, "It's not just that it's bad for you. Do you want to spend the rest of your life fighting a stupid addiction to a stupid thing that doesn't even really give you a good buzz?" — Katherine Heigl

Smoking also hurts you in social situations. It's true that more than half of non-smokers do not like being around smokers. Many people will instantly "un-friend" you if they learn you are a smoker. Just talking to someone with smoker's cough, smoker's breath, and stains on their fingers and teeth is unpleasant. And as the expression goes, "kissing a smoker is like licking out a dirty ashtray." And your nicotine addiction is not cheap; pack-a-day smokers burn more than $40 a week on cigarettes. Most people have much better things to do with their money. Buy something for yourself as a reward for not burning that money up in smoke.

> My dad had emphysema and both of my parents had chronic bronchitis and ended up with cancers - all smoking related. — Loni Anderson

So why did you start smoking in the first place? Years ago we did not know about all the health risks of smoking. Also, to join the group you had to smoke with them. To join the smoke break with your co-workers, you had to smoke. If you didn't smoke you didn't have access to all the latest gossip. In the military, free cigarettes were supplied with your K-rations, and "smoke them if you have them" was a normal part of a work break. The bottom line is that it probably wasn't your fault. But now you realize that you controlled by nicotine and are stuck with an addiction that you need to change.

> The cigarette does the smoking. You're just the sucker.
> — Author unknown

After you finish a cigarette, the nicotine's effects usually lasts for about half an hour. By then, the level of nicotine in your bloodstream drops by about one-half. Soon the nicotine drops even further. You lose your relaxed state and the craving for another cigarette returns. When the nicotine wears off, your body goes through withdrawal, causing agitation, nervousness and uneasiness until you light up again. And when you take the first few puffs of a new cigarette, the withdrawal symptoms quickly disappear and you feel less nervous and more relaxed. So there is a real time correlation between smoking and temporarily feeling better, which reinforces the addictive habit. But remember that the relaxed state is fixing your drug withdrawal. If you were not addicted to nicotine you could have already been relaxed without lighting up. By smoking, you were just getting your addiction fix.

> It is common knowledge that smoking is considered one of the nation's leading causes of preventable death, but it's less widely known that cigarettes are also the leading cause of fatal home fires. — Ed Markey

People are so distracted nowadays that they lose connection with their habit/addiction. They usually think that the cigarette relaxes them, but it was the nicotine withdrawal that made them nervous in the first place. When they feed their addiction they are no longer in withdrawal and they are no longer nervous.

Smoking is a real addiction that is part habit and part chemical dependency. It can be beaten by habit and subconscious mind control because you don't really need a drug to relax. It is the withdrawal from nicotine that made you nervous in the first place, so your body needs more nicotine in order for you to relax.

Nicotine is part on the nightshade family of plants and is a very powerful poison in concentrated form. Just half of a tablespoon of pure nicotine would kill a large grizzly bear. Tobacco plants produce it to kill insects that might feed on the plant. In large doses, nicotine is also a poison for humans and can kill you. Smaller doses act like a stimulus and your heart beats faster. So technically, cigarettes do not relax you. What relaxes you is feeding your nicotine addiction so that you no longer suffer the withdrawal symptoms of the drug.

> They threaten me with lung cancer, and still I smoke and smoke. If they'd only threaten me with hard work, I might stop. — Mignon McLaughlin

The good news is that it is never too late to stop smoking. In just days the damage to your body begins to heal. You will never be totally free of the damage that the cigarettes have caused, but after a few months your body will be considerably healthier and almost back to normal.

> Cigarettes are killers that travel in packs. — Author Unknown

You may think that it is very difficult to stop smoking, and in some situations that's true. If you want to stop just to please someone else then it can be very difficult. If peer pressure or a family member says you should quit, you probably won't. But if you truly want to stop smoking for yourself, and if you follow the instructions in this book, then it is easy to stop smoking.

> Giving up smoking is the easiest thing in the world. I know because I've done it thousands of times. — Mark Twain

Nicotine is one of those drugs in which the first step is to stop smoking long enough so that the withdrawal symptoms are not constantly pressuring you to light up. As with various other drugs, simply cutting down smoking in an attempt to eventually quit will almost always fails. You have to go "cold turkey" (do not smoke even one cigarette) long enough for the drug addiction to stop affecting your body. And that goes for substitutes such as electronic cigarettes and nicotine chewing gum.

Nicotine replacement therapy is useful during the first few weeks of smoking cessation. Those first few weeks when you still have the nicotine addiction are the most uncomfortable period. However many people have enough will power to just quit cold turkey. But this will power probably will not be enough to stop smoking forever.

Nicotine replacements such as nicotine chewing gum, the transdermal nicotine patch, nicotine tablets, nicotine lozenges, nicotine nasal spray and electronic cigarettes do not cure the nicotine addition. All you are doing is changing the drug delivery method. There is some good in this since your lungs are no longer getting that cigarette tar, potassium nitrate, carbon monoxide, various other additives and the many carcinogenic combustion byproducts. But you still get nicotine and nicotine is an insecticide and actually a human poison if taken in large quantities. Replacements also keep you addicted, which means that you will still have to break your addiction. The only positive effect on your ability to actually quit the nicotine addiction is if you use the replacements to make your nicotine withdrawal easier during the difficult first few weeks. Of the various delivery systems, the patch (nicotine transdermal system) is the best one to use because it removes your mouth and hands from your subconscious cigarette habit. Removing the physical makes it easier to stop your addiction. Also there is a regiment to your cutting down your addiction with progressively less powerful patches.

Check with your physician before using the patch,

especially if you have any heart problems, high blood pressure, are pregnant, breast-feeding or taking a prescription medicine for depression or asthma. Follow the directions, which usually say that if you smoke more than half a pack a day to start with the 21 mg patch for a week and then step down to a 14 mg patch and then a 7 mg patch in the following weeks. Some manufacturers will recommend two weeks or more for each step. You must also stop using tobacco or other nicotine products while using the patch. Read the warnings that come with the pack, which typically tell you to stop if you experience symptoms of nicotine overdose such as nausea, vomiting, dizziness, weakness, and rapid heartbeat.

Some people have a skin irritation to the patch. This is generally caused by their allergy to the adhesive in the patch. If you experience this, make sure you apply the patch to a different site every day. Also, you may have to spray or apply a steroid (corticosteroid) on your skin to reduce your allergy.

> A cigarette is the only consumer product which when used as directed kills its consumer. — Dr. George Brundtland

Celebrate each day of being smoke free by putting a large X on your calendar. As the number of X's grows, you will be more and more invested and it will be easier and easier to remain smoke free. Also the visible calendar will strengthen your resolve to be smoke free.

If you are the type of person who likes to be in groups, the odds are definitely better when you try to quit your nicotine addiction with the help of a support group. Your friends and family may offer support, and there are many other more formal support groups. There are also free smartphone quit smoking applications that can help you track your progress toward becoming smoke free. Check out the site at: http://www.smokefree.gov/apps-quitstart.

When you use the information in the next two chapters, your chances of being permanently smoke free are tremendously better.

Trying to cut down on the number of cigarettes you smoke sometimes works but has a poor track record. What happens is that the less you smoke the longer you feel the nicotine withdrawal pains. Then you begin to believe more strongly then ever that you actually do enjoy cigarettes. This of course makes cigarettes seem more important. So often the only thing cutting down does for you is to strengthen your smoking habit.

> Hey, I stopped smoking cigarettes. Isn't that something? I'm on to cigars now. I'm on to a five-year plan. I go to cigars, then I go to pipes, then I go to chewing tobacco, then I'm on to that nicotine gum. — John Candy

Cigarettes are both physically addictive and also psychologically addictive. It is not that hard for most people to stop smoking long enough to temporally kick the nicotine habit. The hard part is the psychological habit that most people do not know how to change and which causes people to start smoking again.

When you first stop smoking it often seems that your cigarette reward is gone and life will be difficult without it. People often feel miserable when they deny themselves the smoking habit that they are dependent upon. They try not to start smoking again, but eventually come to believe that cigarettes are a cherished and pleasurable part of their life. Then they light up and are all the way back at square one.

The missing piece to this puzzle is the habit change that needs to be a major part of permanently kicking the nicotine habit. Fortunately, chapters two and three of this book give you the necessary tools to change your habits so that you will not start smoking again.

I have found that it is best to start your habit change and subconscious mind control (more on those in the following chapters) about a week before you stop smoking. If you use the nicotine patch you can still start the subconscious habit control a week in advance. The reason for this is that the subconscious mind control can be working on the ritual habit of doing something with your hands, lighting a fire and putting something in your mouth to suck.

As babies, one of our prewired habits (instincts) is sucking. A baby's very survival depends on this habit for drinking milk. Sucking comforts and relaxes the baby and soothes any worries. As adults that sucking habit is still wired in our subconscious brain and is a large part of the relaxation we feel when we indulge our smoking habit.

When you stop smoking, or at the conclusion of the patches (usually six or more weeks) you will also have controlled the fire-starting, hand-to-mouth, sucking part of your smoking habit. The main reason so many people fail to permanently stop smoking is because they do not control these rituals inherent to their subconscious smoking habit.

The nicotine patch is available at most drug stores. It is usually available over-the-counter and sometimes also by prescription. Usually you change patches every morning and it delivers nicotine through your skin instead of through your lungs. In most cases, physicians recommend patches of decreasing strength to minimize the nicotine withdrawal symptoms.

> A cigarette is a pipe with a fire at one end and a fool at the other. – Horace Greely

Make your decision about exactly when you will stop smoking, write it down, and stick to it. Pick a specific date to start. Write something to the effect of: On Saturday the 8th of September, I will be smoke free and remain smoke free for the rest of my life. Then sign your name and when the date comes don't let anything stop you.

Your nicotine drug addiction may tell you that because something happened you should postpone your commitment. Do not listen. There is never a good or a bad set of circumstances to become smoke free, so sooner is better than later. Remind yourself of the reasons you want to quit smoking and then just do it.

Habit change and subconscious mind control are key ingredients in your ability to stop smoking. You do not need to bribe yourself with some reward, but you can if you believe it will help. You can control your habits by controlling your subconscious mind. If you follow the directions in chapter two and three your subconscious will obey your wishes. Read the next two chapters to learn how to be the master of your subconscious mind and how to prepare yourself for your new, smoke free life.

Rather than you smoking a cigarette, the cigarette is really smoking you. — Tony Liccione

Some smokers use the excuse that they need to keep smoking to control their weight. It is true that food tastes better and eating gives people something to replace their hand and mouth habit. So some people do find that when they break their addiction, they eat more and gain a few pounds. My advice is to pay attention to your food consumption and weight but do not try to diet while your are quitting your smoking habit. You would be trying to do too much habit change all at the same time. After you beat the nicotine habit is the time you can start working on any weight problems. Other books in the *Conquer and Control* series have sections on overeating and will solve your weight problems. If you do gain weight after you control your smoking, find my weight books at www.conquerandcontrol.com. Most people are able to quit smoking while maintaining their eating habits and do not gain weight.

The believing we do something when we do nothing is the first illusion of tobacco. — Ralph Waldo Emerson

Once you stop smoking for a few months you will find that life is substantially more enjoyable than the misery you encountered when you were addicted. After you stop you must never smoke even a single cigarette again. Remember, it was smoking one cigarette years ago that got you hooked. Even one cigarette could do it again.

Personally, I am what you call an individualist, in that I am generally independent and do not often require a support network. But some people need more group support than others. If your family and friends do not give you the support you need, try Nicotine Anonymous. It is a Non-Profit group whose purpose is to help smokers who want to be smoke free. NA uses the Twelve Step program adapted from Alcoholics Anonymous.

I recommend NA for most people who have an nicotine problem, but it is not for everyone. Here are the three characteristics that can turn certain people off when they go to their first meeting.

1. Nicotine Anonymous is not a religion. However, six of the twelve steps refer to God, Him or a Higher Power. Obviously this will be difficult for you if you are an atheist. However, you could still attend these meetings if you interpret Higher Power or God as your subconscious mind, which you will study in chapter two.

2. In Nicotine Anonymous you are encouraged to tell a large group of strangers your confidential, personal problems, and that may be difficult for you.

3. Some people have difficulty talking in front of groups. However, standing before a sympathetic group of people who share similar suffering due to smoking is a very powerful way to establish a support network for beating your addiction. This is a significant part of the NA method because it combines painful emotions with the emotional support (condolences) and physical support (hugs, handshakes) of a group. You might be able to consider the experience sharing with friends rather than standing in front of a strange group and giving a speech.

If you have any doubts that you can give up cigarettes and be smoke free, drop into one of their group meetings to hear people talk about getting off of nicotine and staying off. Get more information on Nicotine Anonymous at: http://www.nicotine-anonymous.org.

You can see the 12 Steps of Nicotine Anonymous—adapted from Alcoholics Anonymous—on their website at: http://www.nicotine-anonymous.org/publications_content.php?pub_id=18.

I'm glad I don't have to explain to a man from Mars why each day I set fire to dozens of little pieces of paper and put them in my mouth. — Mignon McLaughlin

Chapter Two
Habit Change

Habit is a cable; we weave a thread each day, and at last we cannot break it. — Horace Mann (education reformist)

Humans resist change. Often it takes a disease, crisis or even a tragedy before we take a serious look at who we are and why we are addicted. But right now, you have the opportunity to decide to make the changes that will renew your life.

These next two chapters will give you the insights and techniques you need to change your habits and retake control of your mind. Many thousands of habits—both good and bad—control your everyday life. This book gives you the guidance you have been waiting for to change your negative behaviors.

A habit can be defined as an activity or behavior pattern that we repeat regularly. Habits are keys in our human ability that render us more advanced thinkers than animals. Psychologists also define habits as automatic behaviors triggered by situational cues. Habits make or break us to a far greater extent than we realize. The majority of our everyday actions are controlled by preprogrammed habits, which can either be positive or negative.

The great power of habit for good and bad cannot be overestimated. — Theron Dumont

Habits make our brains more efficient, allowing us to avoid consciously thinking about routine tasks. Instead, we can concentrate on the newer or more challenging aspects of the situation.

Habits also are very important in our ability to perform

tasks quickly and without thinking. A simple example is wearing a seatbelt: most of us buckle up without thinking about it. A more complicated example is riding a bike. Learning to ride a bike requires a lot of attention to balance, and most of us fall a few times in the process of acquiring the skills. But once our subconscious brain takes over and converts a set of actions into an automatic routine, we can ride without ever consciously thinking about balance. Habits can make difficult or complicated things easy.

Habits can also be destructive. They can prevent us from considering why we do something or evaluating if we could do something in a better way. If we engage in a habit over a long enough time period, it becomes a part of who we are, and is therefore that much harder to overcome. You engage in habits subconsciously and often aren't aware that certain actions are actually regulated by a habit. As the saying goes, if you keep doing what you've been doing you'll keep getting what you've got.

Controlling habits is one of the few human skills that are known to produce an extraordinary list of positive benefits in almost all areas of your life. The good news is that you can change any bad habit and get positive benefits.

All of the things that can destroy your life are controlled by powerful habits. Using the instructions in this book, you can take that control back. You may think that willpower is all you need to change bad habits, but that isn't necessarily true. It works for some people, but just using your willpower to stop many habits is very difficult. One of my professors, when talking about willpower and habits, said the average person believes he is above average. In other words, most people think they have above average willpower but in fact their willpower is just average. And most people need stronger than average willpower to change a strong habit.

> What you have to do and the way you have to do it is incredibly simple. Whether you are willing to do it, that's another matter. — Peter F. Drucker

If you think you have enough strength and willpower to stop a strong habit like smoking, then just do it. Many people can temporally stop some bad habits with their willpower. However, most of us are faced with a continuing conflict between the conscious mind that wants to stop smoking and the subconscious mind that wants the smoking habit to repeat itself again and again.

Day after day, month after month, most people will not have enough willpower to constantly fight their craving for smoking. Eventually, while our conscious mind is thinking about something else, some trigger will occur and cause our subconscious to pull us back into that particular bad habit. This could be a vicious circle with temporary victories followed by temporary and eventually long-term failure. Instead of simply trying to control your bad habit with willpower, it is much easier to replace it with a better habit. To do this, you need to understand the operation of habits and the operation of your subconscious mind.

> It's the awareness of how you are stuck that lets you recover.
> — Fritz Perls

Sometimes people are afraid to make changes to their habits. It is the concept of "better to be with the problems I know than those that I do not know". If you have a pet dog you have probably noticed that the dog is happy with its existing habits and does not like any change; at least until it gets accustomed to the new habit.

The good news about the following habit change system is that if you don't like the results you can always use the same old smoking habits you used to have. There is no risk and you have nothing to lose by changing your habit.

> Nothing is impossible. The word itself says, "I'm possible!"
> — Audrey Hepburn

How habits work

The law of habit states that if you repeat an activity enough, it eventually forms a habit. Once the habit is established, your subconscious mind automatically responds in the same way every time a similar cue arises. For people who do not understand the subconscious mind, resisting it often takes more willpower than they have. Trying to fight or resist the habit usually just entrenches it even more strongly. The next chapter will provide more information on the subconscious mind control techniques that you will use to change your unwanted habits.

Pavlov's famous experiment with dogs was one of the first scientific habit experiments that showed the influence of subconscious cues on actions. Pavlov rang a bell as the dogs were given food to eat. Saliva, produced in the mouth, helps in digestion of food. Naturally, the dogs salivated when they saw the food. After a number of bell and food repetitions, the bell was rung without any food but the dogs still salivated. Pavlov discovered that he created a habit in the dogs and the bell alone caused them to salivate.

During childhood, everyone acquires an assortment of various habits that affect them later in life. Some are good, and we want to keep them, but others are bad and negatively affect our lives. These habits are stored deep in our subconscious mind and we often have no awareness of where they first originated.

Like Pavlov's dogs, most of our habits begin without our conscious awareness. We do something and repeat it a number of times and suddenly it is a habit that began without our awareness. For example, one mechanical engineer I know was having difficulties on a project. He felt angry and frustrated, and after work used the whiskey, cheeseburger, and French fry method for coping with the stress. After a couple of months, this cycle became a habit, and he performed this habit every day. Before he knew it, he was overweight and had a drinking problem. He was stuck in this cycle and felt powerless to make a change. He tried again and again to make a change, but he failed every time. He came to believe that he was sentenced to a life of misery and powerless to change. Eventually, he just stopped trying. These types of habits can be very difficult to break using only willpower, but you can change them. Habits can be transformed using the science of habit and mind control described in this book.

> You will be the same person in five years as you are today except for the habits you change.
> — Professor Hal Cohen

In order to change a habit, the first thing you need to do is admit that there is some habit that you want to change. If you smoke three packs of cigarettes a day and still think you are doing it for enjoyment, you will not try to change. In that case, reread the last chapter. If, after reading the smoking chapter, you still think you enjoy your cigarettes, please pass this book on to someone else so they can change their life-destroying habits.

Cue, Action, Reward

> Motivation is what gets you started. Habit is what keeps you going. — Jim Ryun

Habits are created and can be changed with something called the habit cycle. The habit cycle begins with what's called the **cue**, which acts like an icon on your computer screen. When you click the icon, your computer triggers the associated program. It's the same with your brain when something triggers the **cue**. Then your brain turns on the associated routine to begin a particular habit cycle. For example, the smell of someone's cigarette could set off a cue in your mind. A certain song could remind you of a your first love. A certain touch could remind you of your mother's hug. A feeling of frustration, depression, helplessness, and other emotional issues could remind you that a puff on the cigarette will make you feel better. These cues activate habit cycles and were probably setup accidentally and without your conscious awareness. Now they work automatically whenever the cue occurs.

Some cues can be avoided or changed, but some you can't change. When smokers take work breaks, they may be in the habit of smoking during the break. If that is your habit, you will automatically light up whenever you take a break. If your habit is a cigarette after dinner that habit **cue** will be there every time you eat dinner, and we all have to eat.

The habit cycle is as follows:

Cue ➔ Action ➔ Reward ➔➔➔➔ Habit Reset

After the cue comes the **action**, which is triggered by the cue. This is the action you perform. In the case of taking a work break, the action may be to light a cigarette and smoke it. You can't change the cue because you need a break, but can change the action. That is the first key of habit change science. You might find a substitute for smoking such as chewing a stick of gum, eating an apple or contacting a friend on your smart phone.

Finally comes the **reward** where you get a psychological or physical reward. The reward is often receiving some type of desire such as pleasure or social acceptance in the work break group. Similarly, it could be relaxing by avoiding the unpleasantness of nicotine withdrawal. Or it could be the acceptance from your group and avoiding their rejection.

In our after dinner smoke example, you get that comfortable satisfying feeling that comes after a good meal and after smoking. The habit is then reinforced by the reward and reset waiting for the next cue to start the cycle again.

A good way to remember the habit cycle is by using the acronym **CAR**. This stands for **C**ue, **A**ction, and **R**eward. You can think of a car that requires you to steer it. Otherwise, it will steer itself, causing an accident and possibly destroying your life. Habits are the same, and unless we learn how to steer and control them they will control us.

Habits are the foundation of many of our behaviors, and most of them were created subconsciously. Understanding the habit cycle allows us to be aware of these habits and gives us ways of changing them. We can use our understanding to create new routines that will change the habit and eliminate the bad or dangerous consequences of the habit cycle.

The great thing about habits is that once you establish or change them, they become practically effortless. It doesn't matter if you're tired or distracted, or have no willpower; the habit still takes over and fulfills your programming.

> Believe you can and you're halfway there.
> — Theodore Roosevelt

One very powerful key to changing habits is having faith in the possibility that it can be done. Some people might think that changing habits is too theoretical and might not work, but in has in fact worked for many millions of people. If you are dedicated to changing a bad habit, you can trust that this method will work for you just like it has for so many others. Once you understand that we can choose our habits, then you realize that you can succeed in changing them. You can take responsibility for your own life. You can create your own habits.

The thing about habits is you are often unaware they control you. That is why the **CAR** idea is so important. To change a habit, you have to understand how that habit's **C**ue, **A**ction and **R**eward work. It may take some serious contemplation on your part, but the more knowledge you have about the **C**ues, **A**ctions and **R**ewards of your habit, the easier it will be to change them.

Knowledge and purpose are all that is necessary to change a bad habit. Anyone can overcome habits if they truly want to.

I can't change the direction of the wind, but I can adjust my sails to always reach my destination. — Jimmy Dean

Some possible **C**ues that tell people to light up are various smoking paraphernalia. This includes things such as: cigarettes, lighters, matches, and ashtrays. Naturally you will want to remove them from your house and car and definitely throw all your cigarettes in the trashcan.

Other **C**ues involve certain activities such as when you wake up, when you drink alcohol, after sex, when you drink coffee, after a meal, after work. Emotions such as stress, depression, and boredom can also be **C**ues. You can change some of these **C**ues, but usually you can't change all of them (or doing so would be unhealthy, such as in the case of a cigarette after a meal). Here you will have to change the **A**ction or the **R**eward.

Make a list of each **C**ue that makes you want to smoke. Next to each **C**ue write at least one way you can deal with or cope with that **C**ue. Refer to the list while you are detoxing from your smoking habit.

If you can't change the **C**ue, the next easiest link in the **CAR** habit to change is usually the **A**ction. The **R**eward can be changed or modified but is often more difficult.

Sometimes the **C**ue can be modified if you discover that the it is not what it seems. The cue is sometimes more difficult to change since it often comes from our environment. For example, the smells from someone smoking are often just there. Our action may be to get up and investigate the smells and have a smoke. The reward may just be an excuse to take a break from some disagreeable work. If this is the case, you can change the action and instead of a smoke, take a break do something else such as talk to a friend, thereby changing the action and getting basically the same reward of a break but not lighting up a cigarette.

In some cases, the reward might be the temporary relief of your nicotine withdrawal. Removing this reward usually require a period of enforced abstinence to allow your brain the time it needs to rewire itself and break the addiction. Identification of the cue, action and rewards is necessary for the success of the habit change.

You don't need to keep smoking the dangerous nicotine. Nicotine is not calming your nerves but actually just the opposite. Once you are nicotine free for two or three weeks, the nervousness (withdrawal pangs) vanishes and the drug lessens its hold on you. The problem is that you must then change your habits and subconscious mind programming to stay free. Otherwise you will be just like the millions who ride the roller coaster of quit and start and quit and start. So in addition to wanting to quit smoking you can get off the roller coaster if you reprogram your habits using **CAR**, as well as **PREP** and the seven step subconscious habit change sessions, both of which you will learn in the next chapter.

So now it's time to examine your smoking habits. Smoking is an addiction and you feel miserable if you don't smoke, but what are the reasons you tell yourself that you smoke? Usually people will tell me that their reason for smoking is to relieve their anxiety. Others say it helps them concentrate, it gives them a break, it helps them relax, it gives them a lift, it helps their insecurity, et cetera.

As I mentioned, most people have to be nicotine free for about two or three weeks. The reason for this is that the nicotine withdrawal is what sets off your anxiety. This is because the nicotine level in your blood is dropping and your body and subconscious brain are going through withdrawal. It may be difficult for you to believe, but the fact is that the nicotine withdrawal is what makes you anxious. If you never started smoking you would not have this anxiety. This nicotine anxiety will interfere with the **CAR** process, so for you to meaningfully change your smoking habit you must be nicotine free.

It is important to understand the various smoking habits you choose to change. Break the habits down into their cue, action, and reward. Then think about the action and reward, and determine what rewards you are getting from the action you engage in. The next chapter will teach you how to control your subconscious mind. As we go through the following sections on various life-destroying habits, you will learn more about individual habits.

> The greatest things ever done on Earth have been done little by little. — William Bryan

The Japanese have a concept called 'Kaizen.' Kaizen is a series of small steps for continuous improvement of something. Companies such as Toyota use it for quality, technology, productivity and company culture. However, it also works for changing your personal habits.

History has shown us that habit change is most successful when you focus on smaller and more achievable goals. Often you need to break your habit down into small steps. In other words, instead of trying to throw a football the whole hundred yards, take it in baby steps. Throw a series of shorter passes and you still get into the end zone.

> I don't look to jump over 7-foot bars. I look around for 1-foot bars that I can step over. — Warren Buffett

Writers use a similar approach because most people just don't know where to start writing a long book. A large number of writers use the Swiss cheese method, which conceptually starting with a solid piece of cheese and taking out a small piece and then another and another until it is completely gone. Once you start at any point of the cheese, you have your foot in the door and you can move forward with writing your book.

> You don't have to be great to start, but you have to start to be great. — Zig Ziglar

Breaking up a large habit into a number of smaller

habits is an excellent way to overcome your natural resistance to change. Performing a smaller, more manageable habit change still gets you closer to your goal and has other benefits. In addition to beginning your motion towards your large goal it increases your ability to change your habits. It is similar to lifting weights; you start out with a light weight and gradually progress up to heavier ones. With habit change, instead of building muscle, you are building the ability to conquer and control your habits.

If you think small things don't matter, try spending the night in a room with a small mosquito. — Dalai Lama

---

In addition to smoking, you can do this with many other habits such as losing weight. Instead of using all your will power to eat less than 1,000 calories a day, you can just change your habit of eating ice cream for dessert. You can replace the ice cream with an apple. Then a few weeks later after the ice cream habit is successfully changed, you can change another eating habit. The reason this works so well is that learning to change smaller habits rewires you brain and makes it easier to change other habits.

The great value of habits for good and bad cannot be overestimated. Habit is the deepest law of human nature. No one is stronger than their habits, because our habits either build up our strength or decrease it.
— Theron Q. Dumont

Beliefs

Champions don't do extraordinary things. They do ordinary things, but they do them without thinking - too fast for the other team to react. They follow the habits they've learned.
— Tony Dungy, first black coach to win the Super Bowl

The most important thing about changing your habits is your belief that you can do it. An old quote that actually describes how this works is "You must believe it before you see it." In other words, you have to actually believe that the habit will change. If you do not believe it, then it is probable that nothing will change. You must be positive and know you can change. With a negative mindset, you will get negative results. Another saying is "if you believe you can change, you can. But if you believe you can't change, you can't."

There is every reason to believe that you can change any habit. In the real world, every single day, untold thousands of Americans change their bad habits and are no longer controlled by nicotine, alcohol, drugs, over-eating, and all the rest of the major life-destroying habits. These are people from every background and educational level. Smart people can change. Not so smart people can change. Rich people can change. Poor people can change. It doesn't matter everyone is capable of changing their habits. If all of those people can do it, then you can too. It takes some work, but if you are actually motivated to change and believe you can change, then you will. But you have to want it and believe in it. The good news is that through the techniques in this book, it's possible to change old habits and form new ones.

Motivation, belief and the techniques in this book will allow you to bring about your change. The next chapter will provide you with techniques to heighten your will to change. It will explain how your mind works. It will give you techniques to redirect internal narratives so you can control yourself and change habits.

> Winning is not a sometime thing; it's an all time thing.
> Winning is habit. Unfortunately, so is losing.
> — Vince Lombardi

Once you decide which part of your habit you are going to change, write it down. The act of writing gives additional power to your decision to change a habit. Put the note of your decision somewhere prominent, so that you see it every day. You may want to put it on your calendar or in your wallet or purse. In today's world, you can put it on your smart phone or tablet. I put my reminder in my iPad calendar so it appears every day. You should write down the habit change you want in detail in the present tense, as if it were already accomplished. The next chapter will have more information on why you want to write your reminder in the present tense.

Never make an exception to a habit that you recently changed. For example, I changed my habit of always walking down the grocery store candy aisle (and usually buying some candy) to never walking down it. Naturally, a few days later, I had the strongest urge to again walk down this aisle, but my new habit prevailed.

A habit can be thought of as a piece of paper that has been folded. Every time you refold the paper it has a tendency to fold along the same old crease. When we change the habit and make a new crease, the paper will initially easily fold along either the old or the new crease. At that point, a relapse to the old familiar behavioral habit can easily occur. After a week or two of folding in the new direction, the paper has a tendency to fold along the new crease.

You can't always avoid some smoking cues or longings, so make a list of alternative actions you can do to distract yourself for a few minutes. A few of the many possible suggestions are:

Get up and walk somewhere.

Turn on some music.

Phone or text a friend.

Read a magazine or an Internet article.
Go to a smoke free place where you're not allowed to smoke.

> Habit is stronger than reason. — George Santayana

When a business wants its customers to habitually keep coming back, it uses a **CAR** model and adds one other phase to make the habit even more powerful. In addition to the cue, action and reward, they sometimes add investment. For example, if you use Facebook, your investment is in setting up your site with information, pictures and friends. Facebook becomes a powerful habit that will cause you to sign onto your account more often.

Whenever someone starts a risky behavior, whether it's cigarettes, drugs, excessive food, alcohol, or something else entirely, they almost never realize that they are creating a habit and are going to be hooked. If they knew, it is unlikely they would ever smoke that first cigarette and start the habit to begin with. But they didn't believe it would happen to them and now they have a problem. The most effective solution is to change the habit.

> If you don't design your own life plan, chances are you'll fall into someone else's plan. And guess what they have planned for you? Not much. — Jim Rohn

John knew his smokes would be the end of him, but he couldn't stop. He decided not to buy any more cigarettes but every time he ran out there was another carton. He watched a bit of TV and finished another pack.

John's wife knew John needed his smokes to be civil. Without the cigarettes he was an angry and unhappy man. She also believed that the way to a man's heart is to keep him happy. Every time she noticed he was getting short she bought another carton. So John knew he had to fight his habit plus his wife.

John heard about the **CAR** method of habit control and

he knew he had to replace the **A**ction of smoking with something. But nothing seemed to work. John did not know about the **PREP** method you will learn in the next chapter, so he thought that maybe he could change the **C**ue. He had a long talk with his wife and the cartons stopped coming. John cut down on his smokes but he still needed them. Yes, John stumbled and fell back into his addiction, but that wasn't the end. If John knew about the **PREP** method in chapter three and the problems with smoking, he could have changed his habit. Habit change is just the first part of the story; the next part is in chapter three. Below is a flow chart of the **CAR** method that John used. Unfortunately, **CAR** failed, but John now knew he needed something even more powerful. Chapter three has that.

Flow chart of John's process

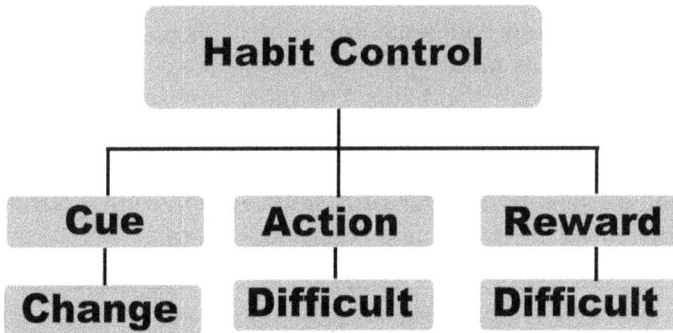

```
                    ┌──────────────────┐
                    │  Habit Control   │
                    └──────────────────┘
            ┌───────────────┼───────────────┐
      ┌──────────┐    ┌──────────┐    ┌──────────┐
      │   Cue    │    │  Action  │    │  Reward  │
      └──────────┘    └──────────┘    └──────────┘
      ┌──────────┐    ┌──────────┐    ┌──────────┐
      │  Change  │    │ Difficult│    │ Difficult│
      └──────────┘    └──────────┘    └──────────┘
```

Summary of Chapter

A habit is something you can do without thinking - which is why most of us have so many of them. — Frank Clark

In this chapter you learned that the vast majority of life is controlled by habits. Nothing is stronger than habits. Most of them are good habits and let you easily accomplish everyday tasks, such as driving a car while thinking of other things. However, some habits are detrimental, and you would like to get rid of them. Often you can just use willpower to delete bad habits, but sometimes you can't. You learned that particularly difficult habits are easier to change than delete. To change a habit, you have to study its components. These components are broken down into **C**ue, **A**ction, and **R**eward, or the acronym '**CAR**.'

There are some destructive habits that are resistant to the power of your conscious decision to change. This is because long-term habits are stored in your subconscious mind. Unless you understand the way your subconscious works it is difficult to consciously change long-term, ingrained habits.

The next chapter focuses on subconscious mind control and will give you important facts about your subconscious mind. It will focus on teaching you methods of talking to your subconscious mind and regaining control of it. You can use your subconscious mind to change one of the components of **CAR** and defeat that bad habit. The most important concepts described in the next chapter are the acronym '**PREP**' and the seven step subconscious session to change habits. With these you will be able to use your conscious mind to change habits that are stored deep in your subconscious mind.

> Sow a thought, and you reap an act. Sow an act, and you reap a habit. Sow a habit, and you reap a character. Sow a character, and you reap a destiny. — Samuel Smiles

CHAPTER THREE
SUBCONSCIOUS MIND CONTROL

> Men occasionally stumble over the truth, but most pick themselves up and hurry off as if nothing has happened.
> — Winston Churchill

Everyone has an unbelievable power, but most people do not know about it. There are numerous things in life you cannot control, but you do have control over yourself and in particular your subconscious mind. You're about to discover the inner workings of your mind and how to control it to your advantage. It will be critical in your habit control, but it will also be important in thousands of other things in your life. You're about to discover how to make your brain's subconscious computer work for you instead of against you. The power to do this is already within you. The simple techniques in this chapter will show you how to use your power and begin a brand new chapter in your life.

The power of your subconscious mind is far greater than you have ever imagined. Your subconscious is where your habits, as well as many other things, are stored. Subconscious mental programming is a wonderful technique that gives you the power to make changes that once seemed impossible. With this technique, you can change your destructive habits and regain control of your life. As you become more familiar with this subconscious technique, you will find that it becomes easier and easier to change all types of habits.

When I was eighteen years old, I took a course in self-defense, taught by a really tough and experienced Korean War Special Forces veteran. In one lesson, I was very surprised how important it is to be aware of how my mind works. The particular lesson I refer to assumed someone was pointing a handgun at me. The trainers asked me what I would say. "Don't shoot", was my immediate response, and the rest of the class nodded in agreement.

"Wrong!" said my trainer. "It is extremely likely that the gunman is operating from his subconscious mind and this mind has difficulty understanding negative words or concepts such as 'don't.' All the subconscious hears is 'shoot.' It is far better to say something positive such as 'You win!' This puts the assailant at ease and removes the pressure from their trigger finger."

Next my trainer showed us how to disarm someone who was within arm's reach. He said, "Before you begin the moves that I will teach you, put the assailant in their conscious mind by asking a question." He recommended after saying, "You win," ask the assailant, "What do you want?" Even though I already knew what the assailant wanted, the purpose of this is to ask a question and cause a delay in the assailant's response time when I start the disarmament move. It turns out that the subconscious responds quickly and reflexively, like a computer or robot. The conscious mind can only think of one thing at a time; it takes a little longer to act because it is weighing the various options of the situation. By contrast, the subconscious mind is much faster. It can think of millions of different things at the same time so it arrives at a solution almost immediately and just does it.

We have two different kinds of minds. The conscious mind can decide which is the best logical course of action, but it is relatively slow. The subconscious mind can intuitively complete previously performed tasks, and it is much faster. You can reprogram your subconscious mind to create better ways to do these tasks.

The subconscious mind is the foundation or our lives because it keeps us alive. It responds to threats much faster than our conscious mind and allows us automatic, split second decisions. It acts to escape dangerous animals or control our automobile to avoid a serious accident. But in addition to keeping us alive, the subconscious mind influences most of our everyday attitudes and decisions on almost everything. As the manager of our many habits, the subconscious mind controls what we eat, what we drink, the drugs we take, and the very health of our bodies. Our ability to regulate our subconscious mind makes all the difference between success and failure in life.

The subconscious mind uses over ninety percent of your brain, while the conscious mind takes less than ten percent. The subconscious mind can do things that the conscious mind has difficulty doing. For example if you are playing tennis and your opponent is winning, you may want to change his subconscious concentration. One way to do this is ask your opponent what he is doing differently to be playing so much better today. If he thinks about it during the next set, he will be in his conscious mind and he may be off his game since he can't react as well or as quickly from his conscious mind. You can try this out yourself by using your conscious mind to think about and do some simple task such as tie your shoe. Your subconscious mind can just do it, but your conscious mind takes longer to figure it out.

I have discovered that the mind behaves as if it had two parts. There is the conscious—or logical, rational—mind, and also the sub-conscious—or irrational, emotional, instinctive—mind. In almost every sport where quick reactions are essential, the good players are those who respond instinctively from the subconscious mind. The conscious mind can control the software that in turn controls the subconscious mind, but if the software did not come from you but was installed by others, the subconscious mind will perform its instructions and override your conscious mind. The physical brain is actually more complicated, but the two minds concept is all you need to know to conquer and control your smoking habits.

In truth, the subconscious mind is the servant of the conscious mind, but it often works in the opposite direction. Your conscious mind often goes to sleep and allows your subconscious to influence the decisions that dictate your life.

Sometimes these decisions cause you to have various addictions that further control your life. When your subconscious mind works against your conscious mind, you will have problems. Unless you know the methods necessary to communicate with your subconscious mind, these problems will control your life.

> By learning the laws of mind, you can extract from that infinite storehouse within you everything you need in order to live life gloriously, joyously, and abundantly.
> — Joseph Murphy

Subconscious Mind

As I indicated, the subconscious mind can process information much more quickly than the conscious mind. When a cornerback intercepts a football pass, his subconscious mind is doing the equivalent of solving hugely complicated equations in just a few seconds. The football's velocity, drop speed, spin and wind direction are just some of the factors. If the linebacker used his conscious mind, the information would not be processed fast enough and there wouldn't be an interception. The linebacker's years of practice in catching passes have forged the action into a subconscious habit and now it just all works automatically.

Many athletes rehearse their moves in their mind while they may be far away from the sports field and possibly even laying in bed. These rehearsals train their subconscious minds to create habits that perform certain actions as a reaction to certain moves by the opposition. Then when they get on to the field, they don't need to engage their conscious mind; the habits in their subconscious mind kick in automatically.

In golf, many top players imagine themselves making perfect swings and visualize the golf ball falling into the hole. These players are in effect changing bad playing habits and replacing them with winning habits. This does not have to be done on the green. Instead, they can practice in their own living rooms using just their minds. Researchers have determined that, even though the muscles do not move, the player's brain waves are identical regardless whether they are on the green or in the living room. When they get on the green, the habits they perfected in their mind magically work to improve their game.

The subconscious mind also takes charge of all the things that happen automatically in your body, such as breathing, digesting food and so forth. While you sleep, it continues to remain alert and even generates your dreams. Additionally, it is an enormous hard drive that records the memories of everything that has happened in your life. It is also the seat of your instincts, emotions, creativity, beliefs and, most relevant to our purposes, your habits. It is the ideal place to make habit changes.

The subconscious remains only in the present time and not in the past or the future. The conscious mind can be in the past, present or future time. So when talking to your subconscious you must stay in the present tense and instead of saying, "I will be brave," you should say, "I am brave."

> Our subconscious minds have no sense of humor, play no jokes, and cannot tell the difference between reality and an imagined thought or image. What we continually think about eventually will manifest in our lives.
> — Robert Collier

The subconscious mind does not normally think with words. Instead, it prefers to use instinctive thoughts such as pictures and emotions. The use of pictures and emotions will allow your subconscious to more readily accept your conscious thoughts and programming. If you try to program the subconscious mind using the wrong words it will reject them. Talking to your subconscious is similar to talking to a three-year-old child; you can't argue with it and you have to talk to it using simple concepts.

Your subconscious can't distinguish between what is

real and what is unreal. No matter how unrealistic a concept is, if you can get your subconscious to believe the idea it will view that concept as a real fact. Then this new belief of your subconscious will be the new normal. And your life will now turn towards the direction of this new normal.

> For one who has conquered the mind, the mind is the best of friends; but for the one who has failed to do so, the mind will remain the greatest enemy. — Bhagavad Gita

As strange as it may seem, your choice of words and thoughts can make all the difference between success and failure with your control of the subconscious. But after you learn the language of your subconscious, you will be able to accomplish anything that you want. You will be able to take control of your life and change the habits that may now be destroying it.

When your subconscious mind accepts any idea, it begins to execute that idea. It is counter-intuitive but true that the subconscious mind accepts both real and unreal ideas equally. It does not argue like your conscious mind would. It is similar to a computer in that whatever it accepts, it believes. With computers, they say "garbage in makes garbage out," and it is the same with your subconscious mind. Our conscious mind sets limits for us, but our subconscious mind has no limits. It can do what we think is impossible. It can change our habits and free us from our addictions.

Many other people and events have already programmed your subconscious mind, but you are mostly unaware of this programming. You have a lot of garbage in your subconscious mind and you are being controlled by events in your childhood environment. It started when you were just a baby and continued through school and beyond. As a young child, your subconscious was aware of most of the things occurring around you, and stored them for future reference. Today, as an adult, this information often affects your thoughts, behaviors and habits. Some of those habits can be very difficult to change if you don't learn the science of how to reprogram your subconscious mind. A prime example is your smoking habit, which you want to change but your subconscious wants to keep.

Your parents or other authorities may have wrongly told you that you were bad at something. That programmed it into your subconscious and to this day you probably still believe it. You were caught up in that belief, but what you didn't understand was that that it was someone else's belief they gave to you. As a child, you had very little choice of what went into your subconscious. Schools, groups, media, and governments continue to exert control of your subconscious habits, with the goal of making you a more manageable subject.

The good news is that your addiction is probably not your fault. Your subconscious mind was programmed by others and it is likely that you had little or no control over the life-destroying habits that resulted. Your addiction is just the normal result of your subconscious mind dealing with various feelings of vulnerability that were programmed into it throughout your life.

The even better news is that habits can be changed, and practically everyone has had to deal with some bad habits at one point in your life. You no longer have to live your life according to the subconscious programming installed when you were too young to realize its consequences. As an adult, you are free to change or at least update the habits that others have installed into your subconscious. This chapter will teach you how to do it.

A man's subconscious self is not the ideal companion. It lurks for the greater part of his life in some dark den of its own, hidden away, and emerges only to taunt and deride and increase the misery of a miserable hour.
—P. G. Wodehouse

The thoughts and images in your conscious mind

become the messages your subconscious believes. Do not continue to think of yourself as a victim controlled by destructive habits that were implanted by others. You have the power to modify what you think, how you feel, and what you do. It is your attitude, and not your prior conditioning, that holds you back from being who you want to be. You can reprogram your subconscious and take control of your life. Make the decision to change the behavior you no longer want.

With the assistance of this book, you can change your addictions, self-image, vulnerabilities, and behaviors that automatically come from your subconscious mind. You can determine the habits that control you and choose to reprogram the undesirable thoughts that were put into your subconscious mind. Using the subconscious mind control methods in this book, you can replace those thoughts with the thoughts you want. You can change your life for the better.

Why be just an average person? All the great achievements of history have been made by strong individuals who refused to consult statistics or to listen to those who could prove convincingly that what they wanted to do, and in fact ultimately did do, was completely impossible.
— Eric Butterworth

Much of your childhood subconscious programming is positive, and you will want to keep it. However, a good deal of it is negative, and this negative programming causes various bad habits and unhealthy states of mind that you will want to change. In order to change a habit, you need to use your conscious brain to reprogram your subconscious brain.

One of mankind's greatest discoveries is that you can alter your life by altering your subconscious mind. The only thing necessary for you to do is learn how to get your subconscious mind to accept your ideas and follow up with the subconscious habit change sessions described at the end of this chapter. Then the power of your subconscious will bring forth the changes you desire.

Any thoughts your subconscious has once learned can be unlearned. However, if you are not intentionally programming your subconscious with the correct thoughts, then it will still be programmed, but the programming will not be in your control and may not be beneficial to you. Understanding your subconscious is essential to successfully programming it.

Do not mistake this subconscious mind programming with simple affirmations. Sometimes affirmations will work, but often the desired habit change does not materialize, even after repeating a statement over and over for months. This is because of weak communication between our subconscious mind and conscious mind. It takes more than just saying some affirmation to make your subconscious believe it is true. You will have to learn the techniques to program your subconscious using the **PREP** method that I will explain later in this chapter.

> Begin to be now what you will be hereafter.
> — William James

To program your subconscious, it is essential that you perform the **PREP** method of subconscious mind control. Once your subconscious is reprogrammed it will faithfully work day and night to bring about the requirements of its programming. If your subconscious is correctly programmed to believe that you should be a certain way, it will make it so. The amount of time that you believed your old programming makes no difference: your new program will take over from your old, obsolete program.

The subconscious mind works 24/7 to control all your body functions. It examines all the sensations (sights, sounds, etc.) coming to you from the outside world and then makes sense of them. It is the center of your emotions and inspirational thoughts. Depending on your subconscious programming, your view of the outside world is most likely different than mine. Unlike your conscious mind, which can only think of one thing at a time, your subconscious can think and do many things at the same time.

Your subconscious mind accepts and believes all thoughts correctly impressed on it by your conscious mind. It is not able to distinguish the difference between truth and untruth. So if you absentmindedly say to yourself, "I'm too dumb" or "I'm too weak" or "I can't do this" and you believe it, then your subconscious will believe you and make sure you are unable to do it. If you tell you subconscious that you just can't seem to stop smoking, you subconscious will believe you and prevent you from quitting. Your subconscious mind will always accept your suggestions and will believe whatever is impressed upon it. It doesn't determine if something is good or bad. It doesn't determine if it is true of false. If you believe and think that you are unable to do something and repeat the thought enough times, then you will not be able to do that thing. Anyone who wants to change their bad habits and grow as a person should learn how to take control of their subconscious mind. When you do this, both your inner and outer worlds will change according to your wishes. If you follow the procedures and instructions of this book you will achieve the habit changes you previously thought to be impossible. But if you do not learn how to control your subconscious mind, then it will control you and your life will be as someone else has programmed. And it may not be to your liking.

When programming your subconscious, think in positives and not negatives. If you are trying to stop smoking, do not focus on giving up or quitting smoking. All quitting thoughts are negatives. Instead, focus on what you want to do and not on what you don't want to do. In other words, you will focus on changing a habit rather than quitting it. You will tell your subconscious that when the habit Cue comes, it will do a different action that produces a different reward--such as chewing gum, for example. Instead of telling your subconscious that you will not smoke any more, use all positives and tell it that you are now smoke free.

Your subconscious mind never sleeps and is always looking after you. Once your subconscious is programmed, when the Cue comes, you will not absentmindedly smoke because your subconscious will be alert and enforce your new habit. Like a computer, it will perform the programmed task, and you will not smoke.

Your subconscious mind does not work in the past or future. It works in the now. Instead of using words such as, "I will do something", use the present tense, which would be, "I do something". Use the present tense and your subconscious will accept you conscious instructions as its fact. Since your subconscious only accepts one concept at a time to be true, it will delete any conflicting beliefs and make your new belief its reality.

What your subconscious mind believes and expects, your life will manifest. This is the key to changing the habits that control your life. An example of this is the placebo effect. During World War Two, my father-in-law was a physician in the Pacific theater of war and often didn't have enough medicine to treat the huge number of causalities. He improvised and gave them a pill he said would ease their pain. Sometimes he even injected them with plain sterile water. Frequently the patient's pain improved despite the fact that the pill was just a placebo (a pill without any medication) with no physical effect on their condition. This happens because the subconscious mind believes that the pill or injection is real. It expects it will help to give them pain relief. Expecting pain relief, the subconscious mind blocks some of the pain.

Another difference between the minds is that the conscious mind tends to be more logical and the subconscious mind is more emotional. The conscious mind is the thinking mind, while the subconscious mind is the feeling mind.

In the province of the mind, what one believes to be true either is true or becomes true. — John Lilly

Conscious Mind

Your consciousness is the logical part of your mind. It can analyze, criticize, judge, and choose between various possible courses of action. You will use your conscious mind to program your subconscious mind. Your subconscious mind has many automatic functions, such as keeping your heart beating and controlling your body's breathing. But in this book, we are not concerned with those functions; se are only concerned with how you can use you conscious mind to program your subconscious mind in order to change your unwanted habits. Your subconscious mind is also the seat of your emotions and the storehouse of memory where your habits are kept. We will use the repetition of emotions and pictures to change the habits performed by your subconscious mind.

If you or your environment conveyed unacceptable habits to your subconscious mind, the surest method of changing them is by communicating positive thoughts— properly directed, of course—to your subconscious. If done properly, your subconscious mind will accept these thoughts, thus forming new and healthy habits.

This is the same thing that many politicians and commercial advertisers do. They use emotions, suggestions, and repetition that your conscious mind may tune out, but your subconscious is always listening and often accepts the message uncritically. The advertisement is not aimed at your critical conscious mind but designed to influence your emotions on a deep, subconscious level. When they repeat the advertisement over and over, your conscious mind tunes it out. But your subconscious is always listening, and when it eventually believes the ad the ad becomes your truth.

In reprogramming your subconscious, it is also often advantageous to include harmonious emotions to give more power to the thoughts you use in programming. You know yourself that when strong emotional things happened to you as a child, you still remember them. Do you remember falling down and hurting yourself when you were learning to ride a bike? How about the time you excelled at something and were publically praised? You remember those things clearly, but you have long since forgotten other less emotional things. So we will often use emotions in addition to positive repetition to change habits more quickly and permanently. If you control your emotional state while you talk to your subconscious mind, you can more easily program it.

You need to understand that you can impress your thoughts upon your subconscious mind to change your habits. You can recreate your life and exchange bad habits for good ones. You can become the person you want to be. A few of us can make these changes using mere self-discipline, but most of us do not yet have that power over our minds. We must use subconscious mind control techniques to change our habitual ways of thinking and to modify the thoughts we no longer want. Eventually, as we have success in our programming, it will become easier and easier.

The law of the subconscious mind is that your programming can be changed by your conscious mind when you apply the procedures shown later in this chapter. You are like a commuter programmer: when you properly program your subconscious mind, it will do your bidding. If you let others program your subconscious mind, it will do their bidding.

One important concept you should accept is that you can change your subconscious thoughts. This change can cause your subconscious mind, and then your entire life, to improve dramatically. You should put aside all other concepts and dwell upon this fact until you have fixed it in your mind.

Do not listen to inner arguments against this idea. If a doubt comes to you, throw it aside. If you take your blinders off, even the darkest night will end and the sun will rise. You absolutely can change your thoughts and your life.

When you accept the power of your ability to control your thoughts, everything changes. It is phenomenal. The entire world seems to change. If weeds were planted in your subconscious mind, you can replace them with flowers. Yes, you can turn lemons into lemonade.

How to Control Your Subconscious

> Before I won my first Mr. Universe, I walked around the tournament like I owned it. I had won it so many times in my mind that there was no doubt I would win it.
> — Arnold Schwarzenegger

When you lose control of your habits and your life, you must redeem them on your own; you will get little encouragement or advice from your friends. Don't expect anyone to help you. Just follow the instructions in this book and resolve to conquer your weaknesses. No one can do this for you. They can encourage you, they can give you examples of others who succeeded, and they can pray for you, but that is all. You must personally follow the procedures outlined in this chapter. You must do the work. Then and only then will you discover that when your habits are changed, new worlds and realities emerge.

> The secret of getting ahead is getting started.
> — Mark Twain

If you want a certain result in your habits, hold the mental image of the result during your subconscious habit change session, which I will soon describe. Keep your conscious mind positively certain that the correct result will come from your effort. Be sure to picture all the details of this result. After forming your thought, have absolute trust that your expectations are now reality. It is not enough that you want to believe it is possible to get a certain result. You must expect the result and know that it is real.

Your conscious mind can weigh ideas and accept or reject them, but your subconscious mind always believes what it is appropriately told. You do not have to prove or argue or fight about the ideas with your subconscious; it just accepts your conscious belief as true. Once your subconscious is programmed and believes something to be true, it controls your life accordingly until it is reprogrammed to believe something else.

The thoughts, pictures and movies you program into your subconscious mind will become reality in your life. You should never think or speak of the change you want in any other way than as being absolutely sure that it is true and is happening. Be positive and your subconscious will accept the desired change as true.

> You can complain because roses have thorns, or you can rejoice because thorns have roses. — Unknown

Your first task to increase your control over your subconscious is to focus on and express your desire of what you want. Do you think it is best to change the **C**ue, the **A**ction or the **R**eward? You have to determine the habit changes you want very clearly and exactly. It should be a very lucid and very real knowledge. You should be able to envision what attaining the change would do for you. See yourself as already having achieved the change. The best place to change the subconscious is with your conscious mind. The **PREP** method shown below is the way to proceed in reprogramming your subconscious mind.

PREP

One of my associates, Bill Malone, came up with the acronym **PREP**. It is a great way to remember the key **Prep**arations necessary to program your subconscious mind.

P is for positive. To program your subconscious mind, you have to send it information in a way that it understands. Your subconscious mind works with positive thoughts, pictures, emotions and feelings. It does not work at all with negative thinking. Remember that your subconscious computer has difficulty with negative words or concepts. It is not as discriminant as the conscious mind and will literally believe anything your conscious mind correctly tells it. The subconscious does not respond well to tentative thoughts such as "possibly" or "maybe". Give it positive, definite information. When I first heard about positive thinking, I thought is was a crock. But when I understood that it could be used as a method to program my subconscious mind, it suddenly made a lot of sense.

R is for repetition. You must repeat the instructions to your subconscious at least once a day for at least two months. This will be described further below.

E is for emotion and energy. Your subconscious mind pays particular value to a concept when you add strong emotions or passions to your programming words. Even advertisers and politicians use energy and emotions to capture your subconscious and get your sale or vote.

P is for picture. You should visualize that you already have the result you want. Think of it not as a change you want, but as a change you already have. Your mental pictures should be very specific and detailed. The more detailed, the better. For example, if you want to be smoke free during a work break, picture yourself as happily talking to your coworkers without a cigarette. You can even turn this picture into a mental movie.

If you want to lose weight, then envision yourself as the body shape that you want, wearing your new clothes. General concepts may not work, so picture yourself exactly as you want to be.

Your conscious mind must portray your desired results, not in the future, but in the present, as if they have already happened. Instead of words like, "I want to," or "I will," use words like, "I am," or "I always." Hold your pictures and thoughts as already being the truth, and your uncritical subconscious will accept them.

The new or changed habit will quickly become your reality. If your conscious mind believes and trusts that you will change then your subconscious mind will also believe that and make it so. Picture your habit as already accomplished. The slogan "fake it until you make it" describes the process perfectly. Accept as fact that the changes you want are already reality. If your conscious mind believes it as fact then soon your subconscious mind will also believe. "Believe it and you will see it," is an expression I heard often during my extensive studies.

Once your subconscious mind accepts your new programming as fact, it will bring this fact into reality and your habit will be changed. You will have reprogrammed your computer and it will now work with you instead of against you.

All belief begins in your will to believe. You cannot always instantaneously believe what you will to believe, but with time and effort your beliefs will change. This must be your first step toward changing your habits.

> The thing always happens that you really believe in and the belief in a thing makes it happen.
> — Frank Lloyd Wright

Your subconscious mind is like a garden, which may be intentionally cultivated or neglected and allowed to grow wild. But whether cultivated or neglected, it will grow. If the seeds are taken randomly from your environment, then an abundance of useless weeds will grow, often resulting in destructive habits. But you can tend the garden of your mind and weed out all the wrong, useless and destructive thoughts, replacing them with the flowers and fruits of useful and constructive thoughts. By pursuing this process you will discovers that you can change bad habits and actually become the director of your life.

A child's conscious mind develops more slowly than their subconscious mind, and habits acquired in childhood color your interpretation of your personal history. Consequently, you have misinterpreted many of the events that occurred in your life. These distorted views of your life's events are now habits which continue to affect you today. For example, some adult may have tried to help by rescuing you from a hole you fell in. But the fall was painful and after the event you associate that particular adult with that pain. The take-away there is that your past memories may not be accurate and, regardless of what you think your past was, you can use habit change and mind control to write your own future. You do not have to go back in time and correct that error; you just have to change your habits in the present time.

Sometimes when you decide to change your life, you might have a fear of failure that could overwhelm your conscious desires. Again, be on guard not to think any negative thoughts lest they be accepted as true by your subconscious. Do not think about your problems, difficulties, or frustrations. Instead imagine your issues are already solved. Picture how the solution looks and how excited and happy you are that they have been solved so quickly.

The subconscious mind responds well to repetition. This is why to program your subconscious mind effectively, you must talk to it every single day. The subconscious will change to your needs if you send it instructions in a way that it understands. Everyone that puts in the effort of working on themselves will be successful.

No matter what you want, envision it clearly with detail. Picture yourself responding in a new way to those smells of food. Add feelings of joy and satisfaction when your changed habits obey your wishes.

The subconscious does not reason or judge how your conscious mind decides the truth. It just accepts and believes everything as factual and right. It works to bring your truth to life. The good news is that you can consciously overcome habits and control and rewrite your subconscious mind to work for you and not against you.

> Nothing great was ever achieved without enthusiasm.
> — Emerson

Set up at least one regular time every day for your

subconscious programming session. This way you make these sessions a routine and then a habit. In the evening just before bedtime or when you first wake up are preferred since at these times your subconscious is most susceptible to thoughts impressed upon it by your conscious mind. Another good time is just before or after a nap. Any regular quiet time of the day can work, but immediately before or after sleep works best. Many people have found that using an event, such as going to bed, works better than just using a clock time. In our busy lives, unexpected occurrences can disrupt our plans for programming at a specific time, but we go to bed virtually every day. The most important thing is to be regular and not to allow any excuse to keep you from your session.

Repeating something often enough causes your subconscious to believe it. This is the reason advertisers show the same commercial over and over.

At the end of your session, be grateful that your new reality is already here. This gratitude is perceived by your subconscious as further proof of what you want, and it will work harder to bring your desires to completion.

> Gratitude makes sense of our past, brings peace for today and creates a vision for tomorrow. — Melody Beatti

Reprogramming your subconscious is similar to building up your muscles at the gym. If you want to lift 300 pounds you might have to start with 30 pounds and work your way up. Training your subconscious is the same: you often have to start with just a part of the total change you eventually want. Every time you consciously reprogram your subconscious it becomes easier and easier.

> The difference between try and triumph is just a little umph! — Marvin Phillips

Seven Step Subconscious Session (SSSS)

Following are the instructions to program your

subconscious mind. In the beginning, it might take you ten minutes or more. With a little practice, it will take seven minutes or less. Everyone who really wants to change a bad habit can find this small amount of time to completely change their life for the better. The best time to do this is just before going to sleep for the night or just after waking up in the morning. The transition between your waking state and your sleeping state naturally allows you better communication with your subconscious mind. Make sure you are in a place where it is unlikely that anything will disrupt your attention.

Seven Step Subconscious Session

Step 1. To begin your Seven Step Subconscious Session, write down the habit you want to change. Use the principles of talking to your subconscious and write it in a present, positive and already true way. If you are working on smoking, an example would be "I am calm, relaxed and smoke free." Because of our formative years in elementary school, our subconscious elevates the written word above other thoughts and accepts it as truth. Handwriting works much better than typing.

Step 2. Sit or lie down, relax, and close your eyes. With your eyes still closed, roll them upward as if you were looking at the top of your forehead. This is an important step that helps your conscious mind communicate with your subconscious.

Step 3. Inhale slowly, deeply drawing air in, and then exhale just as slowly. Let yourself relax as you exhale. Focus your attention on your breathing. Listen to the sound of the air going in and out of your body. Allow yourself to relax as you slowly breath. Do this for three complete breaths. These three deep breaths increase the conscious control of your subconscious mind.

Step 4. Now, with your eyes still closed and still looking upward, speak or think the positive message you wrote down and want to implant into your subconscious. Say "I am calm, relaxed and smoke free."

Change and adjust the words and images to control the

habit of anything you are currently working on. Again, notice the message is in the present tense—"I am"—and not the future tense.

Step 5. Using sensory-rich details, visualize a picture or make a mental movie of your message. See yourself in all the detail you possibly can. Hear the sounds of your coworkers or friends talking. Smell the fresh outside air. Feel the happy thoughts of being smoke free. Try to use as many senses as possible to give substance to your vision. Whatever your goal is, see it as clearly as possible. Make the image crystal clear. Give your vision as much detail as you can. In your first session, there may not be a lot of detail, but as the days go by, you will be able to add more details to your vision.

Step 6. Add emotional content to the positive results. Recall something in your life that made you very happy. This may be a time when you achieved some huge success or some enormous win. It does not matter when it occurred but it must be something that made you feel genuinely happy. Relive the happy emotions of that wonderful past event. Re-experience the good feelings as if they were happening now. Recall your emotions as vividly as you possibly can. Now with those wonderful feelings, continue to repeat your subconscious statements you wrote down from step one.

Step 7. Relax and feel that the picture you created is now an actual fact. See yourself as already owning this habit change. Feel the thrill of your success in altering your habit. This is your new reality, so now open your eyes and give gratitude to the wonderful world that gave you this power. Gratitude is very important, since it signals to your subconscious that you now completed this change, that it is real and is your actual present reality. Your subconscious will then find a way to fulfill this reality.

> Whatever the mind of man can conceive and believe, the mind of man can achieve. — Napoleon Hill

Upon completing your **S**even **S**tep **S**ubconscious

Session, take a minute to examine any ideas you might have had to improve in your next session. For example, your subconscious mind may have given you feedback about something that might give you an insight about a cue, action or reward you are working on. If so, jot it down and adjust your next session to incorporate the new information.

The **S**even **S**tep **S**ubconscious **S**ession has linked happy feelings with change images and implanted them directly into your subconscious mind. This will cause your old habit to be replaced with your new visions. But one session is definitely not enough. Your old habit may have been in control for years and years, so it will take time to permanently change it. You have to be prepared to repeat these sessions for about two months. Everyone's time varies—some people can change a habit in a few weeks, while for others it may take six months. It also depends on the particular habit and your experience in habit change. If this is your first try, it may take longer. Additionally, a very strong habit will definitely take longer than a weak habit. As explained in the first chapter, you will need to detox your body so that the nicotine drug does not interfere with your **SSSS**, so changing your smoking habit will definitely be one of the longer processes. Don't be discouraged, though; with patience and dedication, you can completely turn the habit around.

Notice that in this example, we used a **P**ositive statement, "I am calm, relaxed and smoke free" instead of, "I will stop smoking". The **R**epetition is daily for about a month or more. The **E**motion is to recall something in your life that made you very happy. And the **P**icture is to see the eventual results as your present reality. See the lack of a cigarette in all the detail you possibly can. You can also include hearing and feeling senses. Your mental pictures should be very detailed; the more the better. It can even be a mental movie.

The methods here are for people whose desire for change is strong enough to overcome laziness and do the **S**even **S**tep **S**ubconscious **S**ession. A daily commitment is necessary. With this commitment, you must have an unwavering faith (fake it till you make it) that the habit is already changed and all you have to do is recognize it. Repetition is the key.

Again, what you have to do is form a distinct mental image of the goal you want. The goal comes from the habit you are changing. Also, hold fast to your purpose and be positive that your results will be forthcoming. Even if at first it takes more than two months, keep your positive attitude; if you do not believe, then your subconscious mind will not believe and it will resist change.

There is no chance, no destiny, no fate that can circumvent or hinder or control the firm resolve of a determined soul.
— Ella Wheeler Wilcox

Things that dominate our thoughts also dominate our beliefs. If you want to become sober, you most likely shouldn't make a study of types of wine and bourbon. Also, things are not brought into reality by thinking about their opposites.

Doubt or unbelief is as certain to start a movement away from your goals as faith and purpose are to start one toward them. Every minute you spend giving power to doubts and fears, every minute you spend in worry, every minute in which you are possessed by unbelief sets a current away from your goal of changing your habits.

Destiny is not a matter of chance, it is a matter of choice; it is not a thing to be waited for. It is a thing to be achieved.
— Winston Churchill

If you look at the majority of advertising and political campaigns that are directed at you, you will notice that very few of them use conscious, logical reasoning. They mostly use dumb advertisements that are filled with suggestions, dreams, emotions and images that are implanted directly into your subconscious mind without any critical listening from your conscious mind. They have found that talking to your subconscious works and they spend many billions of dollars doing it. It works for them, and it will also work for you when you use the principles in this chapter.

Do not argue with your subconscious. Remember that your subconscious is like a computer. You do not argue with your computer program. You know that your computer will not do something it was not programmed to do; you have to update the programming to get the functions you desire. It is the same with your subconscious.

> What lies behind us, and what lies before us are small matters compared to what lies within us.
> — Ralph Waldo Emerson

Use the instructions in this chapter to control your subconscious. Repeat the **SSSS** exercise once or twice a day. These seven steps may seem strange to you, but our subconscious mind is strange. We can either control it or it will control us. I choose control over my subconscious, and I hope you choose the same.

Your subconscious believes that there is something more official and real in the written word. In step one of the **S**even **S**tep **S**ubconscious **S**ession, you wrote down the habit you want to change as if it were already accomplished. Keep this paper in your wallet or purse until this habit change is established.

Computers and smart phones now have a number of programs that track and assist in forming habits. I believe that paper and pen work better, but some people prefer doing it digitally. If you are one of those people, do some research and find an app that works for you.

> There is a tide in the affairs of men, which, taken at the flood leads on to fortune. Omitted, all the voyage of their life is bound in shallows and in miseries.
> — William Shakespeare

You may think that change in your life should happen in the way that you expect, but often it's the opposite. You may try to change one part of your habit in a certain way but find that another part changed. Regardless of the exact change, your bad habit will have been fixed. Do not be concerned about how things arrive; instead, hold onto your vision and follow the principles of subconscious mind control, and everything will end up in its place.

The power of belief is fantastic. For all of recorded history, it was believed that humans were physically unable to run a four-minute mile. No one did until 1954. Then along came Roger Bannister, who not only believed it could be done but actually did it. The amazing thing, however, is that once people realized that four minutes was not a physical barrier but just a subconscious belief, everything changed. Within the next year, thirty other people had also ran a four-minute mile. Before 1954, no one could. By 1955, 31 people had.

For difficult habits, it sometimes helps to tell someone or some group about the change in your life. This is especially true for social people who are usually in groups or on their smart phones instead of by themselves. But never share your habit change progress with envious or negative people. Your subconscious will hear their negative response and possibly believe it. Only share your progress with positive, supportive people who will encourage you to continue your quest to conquer and control your habits.

> There is a track just waiting there for each of us, and once on it, doors will open that were not open before and would not open for anyone else. — Joseph Campbell

Most people are controlled by their subconscious and driven by the insecurities, vulnerabilities and inadequacies in their life. They are passengers on the road of life and not drivers of the car. If you're not in the driving seat, you're being controlled or subjugated by the mental programs that you accepted without even knowing it. You don't have to be subjugated by the mindless conditions that would rule and control you. If you use your conscious mind to reprogram your subconscious mind, you will no longer allow people or conditions to take advantage of you.

We all have worldly desires, and the subconscious directs us to do whatever it takes to fulfill these desires. You can rise above the programming and be free to choose your destiny.

Yes, it's easier to just go along with the crowd and do what they're doing, but you'll end up like they are. You will be subjugated. You will be one of the masses, a cog in the wheel, a digit in a computer.

Psychology and money are the two main tools that people use to control you. But you don't need approval from others if it results in their control. Also, you don't need conventional status symbols, such as a million dollars or the finest sports car.

> Laugh and the world laughs with you; cry and you cry alone.
> — Unknown

A study was performed to demonstrate how controlled we are by social norms. The participants were divided into three groups. Group one was told that they would hear a joke and to behave as if it was a great joke. Groups two and three were not told anything. Groups one and two were put back together and after hearing a really bad joke group one laughed as they were told, and many in group two also began giggling and feeling surprisingly euphoric. As a control, group one was then told next time not to laugh at the joke. Groups one and three were put together and and the same bad joke was told. No one laughed and the joke bombed. It was the same joke but no one in group three laughed or thought it was a good joke. This is the same concept as the laugh track often played on TV comedy shows where the laughing from the TV show causes many viewers to be more prone to laugh.

You can use this concept by yourself. Your behavior can create your emotions which are useful in the habit change exercise. Purposely tell yourself to smile and you feel happier. Tense your muscles and pretend that you are vulnerable and in danger, and you become uptight and more focused on the present moment.

> It is never too late to be what you might have been.
> — George Eliot

I remember when I was young, a huge football player had words with me. Then he made a fist and took a swing at me. My subconscious mind took over and all I did was perform a very small action than had previously become a habit due to my training over and over in this precise move. I instinctively parried and, keeping contact with his arm, I pulled it. At the same time, I took a small step backward. He was off-balance due to the force of his swing, and I pulled him forward down hard. He hit the concrete ground with a very loud thump. He knocked himself out and didn't move. I looked around and saw he had a few friends, so I made a very quick exit. Due to many hundreds of repetitions, that one small step and pull became a habit in my subconscious mind and it saved me from what might have been a very dangerous situation.

If you are just starting out with habit control and trying to make a huge change, but have difficulty changing your habits, then take them one small step at a time. Just the smallest actions can make a big difference in your life. You don't have to go for the home run; just get on base.

> Nothing is particularly hard if you divide it into small jobs.
> — Henry Ford

In China, there is an old saying that "a journey of a thousand miles starts with a single step." Steve Jobs used this concept with his computers, iPods, iPads and iPhones. He came out with a great product and continued to improve the original model making it better and better.

Often, changing a big habit seems overpowering, so the solution is to break the habit down into a number of smaller changes. This develops the awareness that change is possible and strengthens your habit control. As you see the success of this concept, move ahead and change other habits until you complete all the changes you want.

> The great thing in the world is not so much where we stand as in what direction we are moving.
> — Oliver Wendell Holmes

After you change your unwanted smoking habit, you may find that the psychological emotions your habit covered up are now exposed. It is good to pay attention to these exposed emotions because this gives you an opportunity for a deeper understanding of what issues drove your unwanted habit. Some people have found that these exposed emotions are redirected into other areas of their life. Fortunately, subconscious mind programming is also effective in eliminating the underlying issues and emotions that drove your habits in the first place. Alternatively, you may want to consult a professional to assist you with these issues.

Often times there are social habits that reinforce addictions. For example, if your social life revolves around a group where everyone smokes you will need to change your social life and the places you frequent. Fortunately, subconscious mind programming works on this as well as the nicotine addictions.

> Habit is habit, not to be thrown out the window by any man, but rather coaxed down the stairs one step at a time.
> — Mark Twain

Addictions are habits that are often associated with underlying emotions stored in your subconscious mind. Traumas, childhood abuse, neglect, violence, vulnerability and emotional distress are some of the occurrences that produce these destructive habits. This is why we reprogram the subconscious and change these unwanted habits.

> Knowing is not enough. We must apply. Willing is not enough. We must do. — Johann Goethe

Summary of the Chapter

The only thing that could stop you from realizing the dream of changing your life-destroying smoking habit is procrastination. Procrastination means putting off something that you know you should do because of fear of change, avoiding confrontations, avoiding responsibility or some other belief or feeling that drives you to maintain the status quo.

I am here to tell you that the habit change technology from chapter two combined with the subconscious mind control in this chapter is almost magic. It will lift your life to the next level where you will be free of the smoking habits that are slowly killing you. The only real thing that keeps you from taking action is you. You owe it to yourself to move beyond procrastination and take control of your life.

> I've failed over and over and over again in my life, and that is why I succeed. — Michael Jordan

Jane had a difficult boss at work, and every day he criticized her. One of her coworkers was laid off and Jane was expected to take up the slack. Jane felt helpless and could barely make it through the day. She thought about quitting and getting another job, but it was a difficult job market, the economy was bad and her pay was good. She knew that she was helplessly trapped. So to relax, she smoked almost two packs of cigarettes. They temporally took her mind off her problems and made Jane feel better, but she was coughing a lot and knew she had to change her habits.

Jane examined the **CAR** of her habit and knew her boss

wouldn't change so the **C**ue would be difficult to change. She also knew she needed some reward after work to make up for that terrible boss. So that left the **A**ction as the best bet to change. Her husband's health club had a Precore elliptical machine, so on the way home she stopped in and used it for half an hour. It worked and she was able to skip the cigarettes and take her anger and frustration out on the machine. On one unusually difficult day, however, her old **CAR** automatically drove her back to her old smoking habit.

Jane knew it was time to use the **PREP** method to permanently change her action regarding those smokes. So for **P**ositive she decided on, "To relax after work, I use the elliptical machine." For **R**epetition, she used every evening while lying in bed just before she went to sleep. Because of her anger at work, the **E**motions were easy. She just imagined that peace and serenity surrounded her when she walked on the machine. Finally, for the **P**icture, she envisioned herself as if in a movie, exercising on the elliptical machine and relaxing into a peaceful state.

She used this movie in her **S**even **S**tep **S**ubconscious **S**ession. First she wrote down that after work, she would use her elliptical machine to relax. Then every night as she was falling asleep, she rolled her eyes upward and slowly took seven breaths. She spoke the words she wrote on the paper and envisioned herself using the elliptical machine while being in a relaxed, peaceful state. She recalled the joy she felt when her father taught her to ride a bike and saw her actions as real and true. Then she gave thanks for the peace and comfort the elliptical machine gave her. In the days that followed, the old smoking habit was magically and permanently changed into the exercise habit.

Flow chart of Jane's process

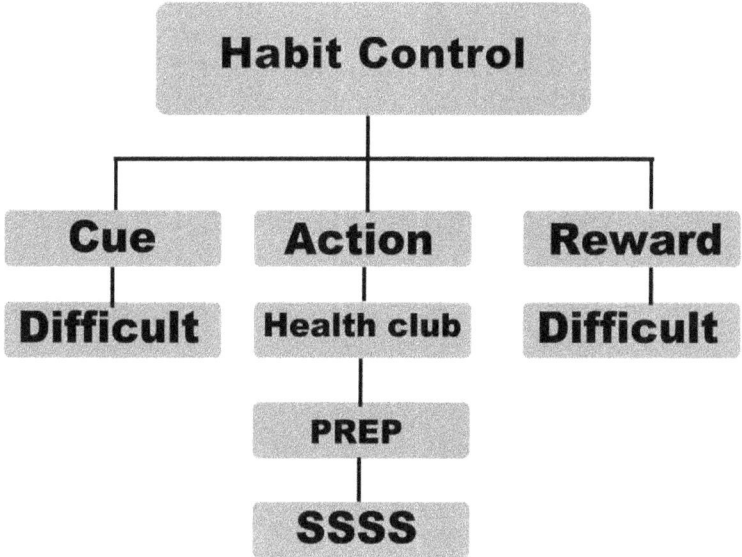

Habit Control

Cue	Action	Reward
Difficult	**Health club**	**Difficult**
	PREP	
	SSSS	

In this chapter, we learned the **PREP** technology. You can use **PREP** to change one of the components of **CAR** (from the previous chapter) and defeat the habit that is destroying your life.

<u>P is for positive</u>. Your subconscious computer has difficulty with negative words or concepts.
<u>R is for repetition</u>. You must repeat the instructions to your subconscious at least twice a day for at least a month or two.
<u>E is for emotion</u>. Your subconscious mind places particular value on a concept when you add strong emotions or passions to your programming words.
<u>P is for picture</u>. Your mental pictures should be very detailed. The more detailed the better.

"Fake it until you make it," is an easy to remember slogan that describes the concept. Accept as fact that the changes you want are already reality. If your conscious mind believes it, then soon your subconscious will also believe. Once your subconscious accepts your new programming as fact, it will make that fact reality and your habit will be changed. You will have reprogrammed your computer, and it will now work with you instead of against you.

Do not be overly alarmed if you have a few relapses into your previous habit pattern. Just continue to faithfully do your subconscious mind reprogramming and you will soon be completely successful.

CONCLUSION

Your resistance to change is likely to reach its peak when significant change is imminent. — George Leonard

In chapter two you learned that a habit is a **C**ue, an **A**ction and a **R**eward. Many habits can be changed by just changing one of these three components. Often your willpower and the knowledge of how habits work is all you need.

However, smoking habits are difficult for most people to change with just willpower. Your conscious mind controls your willpower. If you decide to stop smoking by relying solely on willpower, you could easily fail. This is because in addition to your nicotine addiction, your other smoking habits are stored in your subconscious mind, which is stronger than your conscious mind. After a few weeks your willpower may wane and if you have a weak moment, you can easily light up a cigarette and begin you addiction anew. Habits are stored in your subconscious mind, and it is easiest to change them there.

To reprogram the subconscious, you need to know how to communicate with it. You learned to use **PREP** which stands for **P**ositive, **R**epetition, **E**motion and **P**ictures. Then you learned how to perform your daily subconscious mind programming called the **S**even **S**tep **S**ubconscious **S**ystem.

In this book, I focused on smoking habits. However, there are literally thousands of additional habits that you may want to change. The **CAR**, **PREP**, and **SSSS** instructions will allow you to change them.

My big book _Conquer and Control Your Habits and Your Life_ shows you how to change many other habits using similar techniques. It is the big book from which much of this book you are reading was taken.

Some of these habits are certainly minor, but you can

still change them. For example, my physician told me to cut down my coffee drinking to eliminate my stomach pains. I easily went from eight cups a day down to just one. I probably could have done this with willpower, but it was easier to just let my subconscious mind take care of it.

> In any family, measles are less contagious than bad habits.
> — Mignon McLaughlin

If you are a student, you can change your study habits. If you fear public speaking, you can change that habit. The possibilities are endless. In the future, I will have more detailed information on changing some of these less critical habits. The web site http://www.conquerandcontrol.com will examine changing more peripheral habits.

Subconscious programming can also be used to switch off various abnormalities that cause pain. However, you should first consult your physician, because pain can be an indicator of a disease that requires treatment.

ABOUT THE AUTHOR

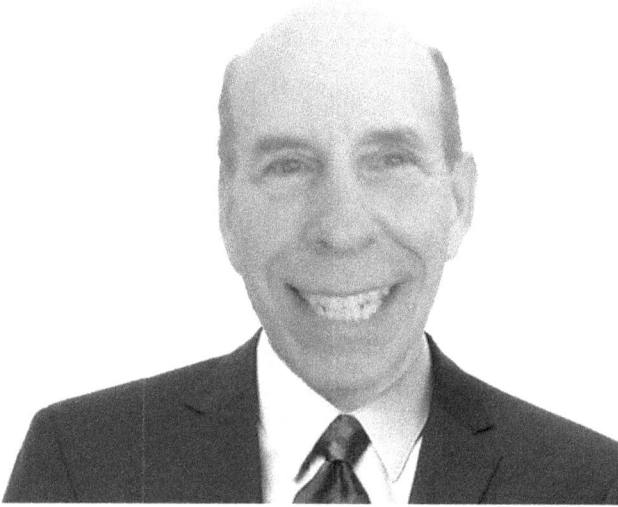

Alan Fensin began his career with Boeing and NASA in the early days of the American space program. He was a key member of the Apollo rocket design team that successfully put a man on the moon. As an electrical engineer, Alan helped design many of the critical elements used in the electrical system of the Saturn 5 moon–rocket. Returning to school in 1976, he earned an MBA from Tulane University, majoring in Behavior Analysis.

During the early 1990's, he discovered the *Conquer and Control* concepts and this system for using the subconscious mind to change unwanted habits. He believes that this knowledge changed his life, exposing and dealing with problems that had previously limited his growth.

He has been a lecturer and writer for the last twenty years.